Dreams

100 Affirmations for a Good Night's Sleep

Elicia Rose

ROCK
POINT
QUARTOKNOWS.COM
NEW YORK, NY

Thank you to Lizzie and Sophie:
your friendship means the
world to me.

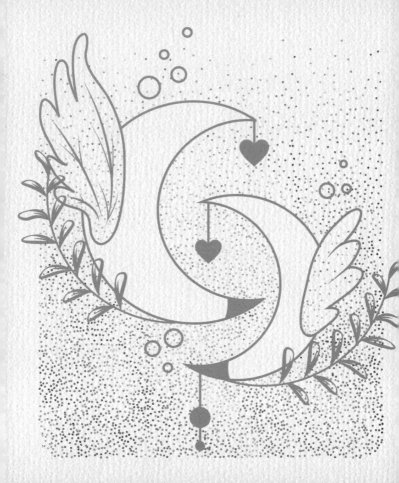

Contents

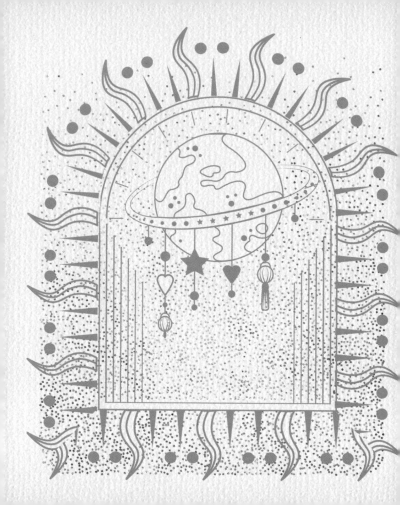

Introduction

We all know how much better we feel after a good night's sleep. The day seems to flow easier, conversations with loved ones are more harmonious, and the little things that might usually throw us off don't have as much of an impact. Being able to switch off and allow the body to do its thing should be the most natural process in the world, yet why do so many of us struggle to wake up feeling refreshed?

In recent years, sleep issues such as insomnia, restlessness, and a whole host of other problems have risen on a global scale. We now know the dangers of not sleeping properly, affecting everything from energy levels to cognitive function. Despite knowing the benefits of sleeping properly, many of us still can't sleep well, no matter how hard we try. In this book, you'll find affirmations, reflections, and exercises, all centered around helping you attain a good night's sleep by examining your mind-set, current habits, and the pressure you put on yourself to sleep well.

I believe our ability to sleep well is directly linked to our ability to rest, relax, and switch off from the outside world, which, let's face it, is more and more difficult with the demands that society places on us. When our minds are constantly on overdrive, we struggle to fully let go and rest deeply. I also believe it's helpful to examine our current beliefs around being worthy of deep, replenishing rest and sleep. If, deep down, you believe you don't deserve to put your needs first and prioritize self-care, then a full eight hours in bed might seem like a luxury, rather than a necessity.

No matter how hard we try, it is impossible to predict the future and know everything that is going to occur, whether good or bad. There will be phases of life where a good night's sleep just isn't possible. Rather than increasing levels of stress (which will already be increased due to a lack of sleep), I offer another solution: to make peace with the unpredictable nature of life. Some nights we will sleep soundly, and some nights this won't be possible, and that is okay. Learning to make peace with what is going on in our lives is a great way to enhance feelings of calm.

I discovered positive affirmations while studying at the university. As I moved to a new city and experienced a lot of changes in a short amount of time, I noticed

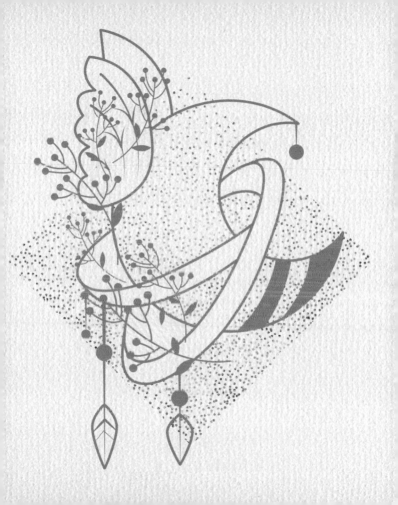

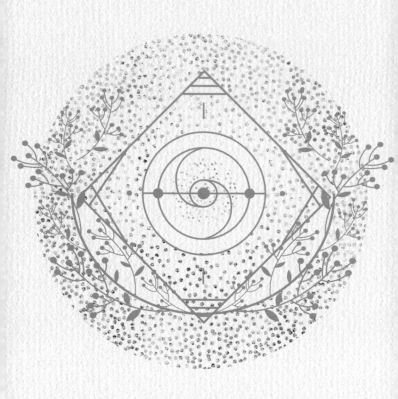

negative and unhelpful thoughts begin to creep in. Rather than listen to these thoughts, I began to speak, think, and journal statements that were much more helpful. I couldn't believe how quickly they worked. I realized that if they could help me feel better about myself, then they definitely had the power to help others feel better about themselves too, in any area of life, which was when my idea for my business Bloom Affirmations started. We are what we repeatedly tell ourselves, so this book will help you take back control of the way you think.

Affirmations offer a powerful tool to help us rewire the conscious and subconscious parts of our mind, challenging the negative or unhelpful beliefs we might have picked up. The key here is repetition.

Speak your affirmations aloud, write them in your journal, and put them in places where you'll notice them throughout the day. Use the reflections and exercises to further develop your self-awareness around what you currently think and feel. The affirmations, reflections, and exercises in this book may not be the full solution to attaining a good night's sleep, but they will certainly help you embrace a healthier mind-set and cultivate deep inner peace.

No matter how busy your life is and how many demands you face on a daily basis, know that sleep and rest are important. They are essential to every single body function and allow us to enjoy life to the fullest. You are absolutely worthy of a good night's sleep, and you absolutely can make positive and lasting changes that support this.

You can read this book in order, or you can choose a page at random for a daily focus. Take your time with each affirmation, reflection, and exercise, and be gentle with yourself.

Affirmations aren't the full solution to helping you sleep better, but my hope is that as you read this book, you'll begin to develop an awareness of what is stopping you from resting fully. If you notice that a particular affirmation, meditation, or journal prompt creates resistance within you, I invite you to explore the reasons behind this. When we are willing to look at what triggers us with an open and inquisitive mind, we might just learn a very important lesson. You might even wish to keep a separate journal as you work through this book to note any interesting thoughts and feelings.

The journey to becoming a grounded and more balanced person doesn't need to be intense; even five minutes a day of doing something that brings you peace can have a transformative effect. Be proud of yourself for wanting to make positive changes and enjoy the journey for deeper rest.

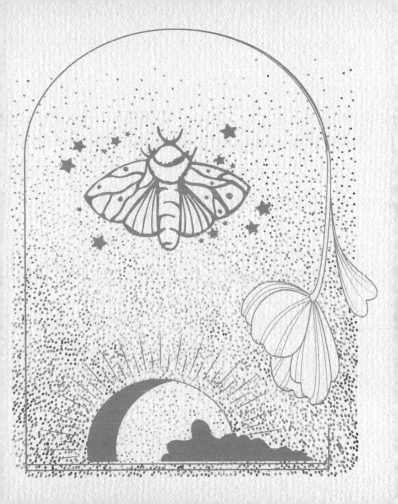

Worthiness

I n order to promote a good night's sleep, it's important to examine your thoughts and beliefs about feeling worthy of deep rest and relaxation. If you don't believe your needs are important, then it's likely you will spend more time prioritizing other commitments rather than looking after yourself, which is a quick path to feeling burned out and overwhelmed.

Self-care is vital for our overall well-being, and sleep is one of the best ways that we can take care of ourselves. As the famous saying goes, you can't pour from an empty cup. The better you feel within yourself, the more you have to offer to all areas of your life, and feeling better within yourself often begins with making sure your needs are taken care of.

We all have different schedules and paces of life, but I promise you, it is always possible to find the time to practice some form of self-care. Even if you only have ten minutes to yourself, you can still find the time to do something that helps replenish your cup.

The following affirmations and exercises are designed to explore your current beliefs about rest and relaxation and increase feelings of worthiness around taking the time to tend to your needs.

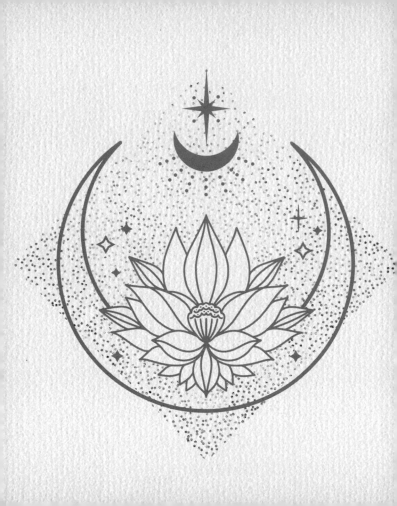

I am worthy of deep rest and relaxation

You are always worthy of deep rest and relaxation. You don't need to do anything to earn it, and you don't need to prove to anyone else why you deserve to look after yourself.

Complete this sentence: I choose to prioritize deep rest and relaxation because . . .

I deserve to feel rested and revitalized

Intentionally make some time this week to get more rest and give yourself the time to unwind. This can be taking a few extra minutes to stay in bed, taking a few extra seconds to meditate, or remembering to sit down and take a break. To feel revitalized, it's important to give yourself the space to fully rest.

What is one activity or practice that makes you feel completely rested?

I release any resistance around prioritizing my needs

It's normal to experience resistance around prioritizing your needs, especially if you're so out of touch with them. It helps to journal about your current priorities to gain an understanding on how self-care fits into this.

Think about your top priorities in life. Where does taking care of yourself fit in? If it doesn't rank as high as you'd like it to, what are the reasons for this and what can you do to change this? It's common to view self-care as self-indulgent, but in reality, self-care isn't about treating yourself to a massage every week (although if that's how you like to take care of yourself, then go ahead!). It's about giving yourself that extra time and space you need to feel restored, even if it's just five minutes of alone time.

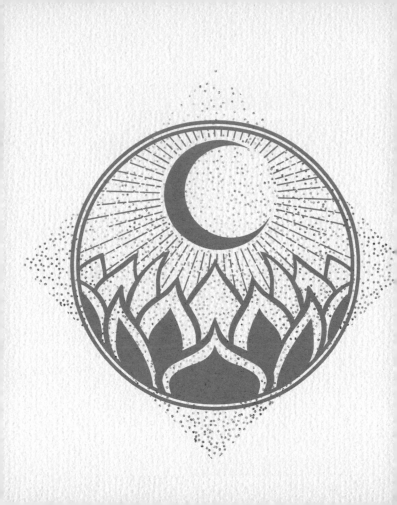

I can take care of myself and still take care of others

Taking care of yourself does not mean that you have to stop looking after others. You can still make time for both, and the more you take care of yourself, the more you'll have to offer others.

Do you believe it is possible to look after your own needs as well as the needs of others? If the answer is no, explore in your journal where you might have learned this from.

I make time for self-care and relaxation

Holding the belief that self-care is important is very different to actually making time for it and taking physical actions to make it a priority.

If you lead a busy life, schedule something completely relaxing and restorative and put it in your calendar. Turn this into a weekly habit if possible. It doesn't have to be a whole day or evening—even half an hour or a few minutes will still be effective.

I love myself, and I value my own needs

When was the last time you stopped and considered yourself as someone who is valuable, worthy, and deserving of care?

Complete this sentence: I am worthy of taking care of myself because . . .

I am worthy exactly as I am

You can strive to make positive changes and improve your life while also holding the belief that you are worthy exactly as you are. Making changes from this place means you are making them for the right reasons.

Try this mirror affirmation exercise. Repeat the affirmation on this page aloud to yourself while looking in the mirror. Keep repeating the affirmation as you look into your own eyes, placing your hands over your heart if you wish.

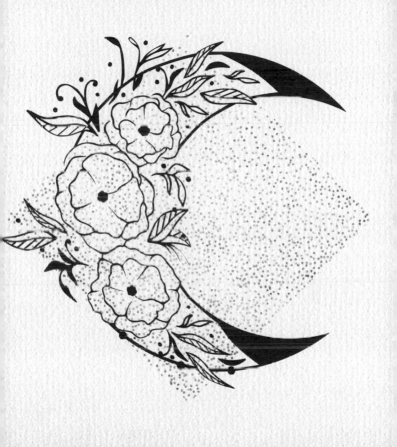

I understand the importance of rest

Every single part of nature takes time to slow down and recuperate. Flowers don't bloom all year round, many animals hibernate in the winter, and even the sun sets every day. You are part of nature, and therefore you also need to take time to slow down and rest.

Make a list of all the reasons why rest is important to you.

I nurture feelings of worthiness toward myself

You might have experienced things that have made you feel unworthy or unlovable. Now it's time to release these stories.

Practice this self-soothing meditation. Find a comfortable position where you won't be disturbed and close your eyes. Turn your attention to your breathing. Begin to breathe deeper and slower. As you begin to settle, wrap your arms around yourself and give yourself a big hug. Keep breathing deeply and receive your own love. Know that you will always be there to support yourself.

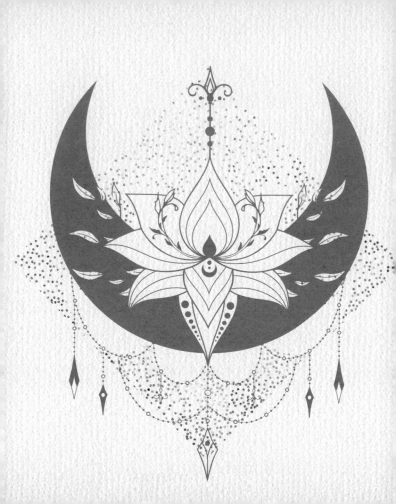

Today I choose to be true to myself and honor my needs

Your needs are very important, and you deserve to meet them. Similarly, expressing your needs and their importance to others is the basis of a healthy and thriving relationship.

What is one need you have been neglecting recently? Why have you been neglecting it? What is one action you can take to help address this need?

I let go of any limiting beliefs and replace them with love and acceptance

It is completely within your power to let worries float away and invite more loving and supportive thoughts into your mind.

Make a list of the limiting beliefs you have around looking after yourself. Include all the negativity, fear, or doubts. Once you have written this list, cross out each reason and replace it with a more encouraging or helpful statement. An example might be turning "I'm too busy and I don't have the time" to "I am willing to make the time to look after myself, even if I start small."

My needs are important, and I deserve to have them met

When you first begin identifying your own needs, it's a good idea to start meeting the ones you are in control of. As you get comfortable addressing your own needs, you can then begin expressing the ones that require input from others.

Make a list of the needs you can meet yourself on a daily or weekly basis. Do they require planning, clearing space in your calendar, or any other changes to accommodate them?

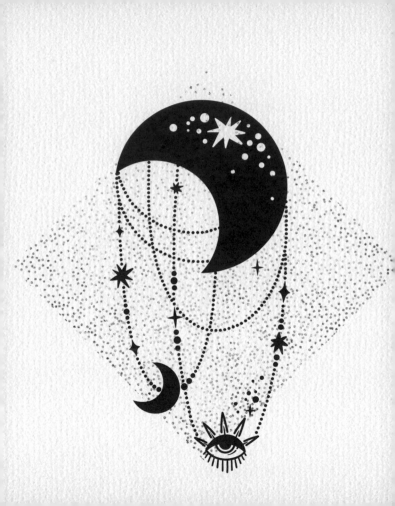

The more I rest, the more I have to offer

It is difficult to offer more to other areas of your life, including your loved ones, if you don't feel rested yourself.

Choose one relationship that means a lot to you and journal all the ways this relationship would benefit if you decided to take care of your needs first. You might want to share this list with the person and encourage them to create their own list.

I already know what works and doesn't work for me

Everyone requires a different amount of sleep and varying sleep conditions to wake up feeling good.

What would a good night's sleep look like to you? What time would you go to bed and what time would you wake up? How many hours of sleep would you get? How would you feel when you wake up in the morning?

My existence is valuable. I am inherently worthy

You don't need to do anything in order to be worthy. You are worthy exactly as you are, and so is every other human. Read that again. You might receive messages on a daily basis that you need to be, do, and have more, but the reality is your worthiness is not dependent on any external circumstance.

Write the above affirmation in your journal at least three times. Allow the power of these words to sink in. Return to this affirmation whenever you feel self-doubt or judgment.

I am willing to invite more self-care into my life

Self-care might seem like an abstract concept, so take some time to reflect on what it means to you and how you'd like it to show up in your life.

What are your favorite forms of self-care? Make a list of all the ways you like to take care of yourself and the activities that make you feel nourished and restored.

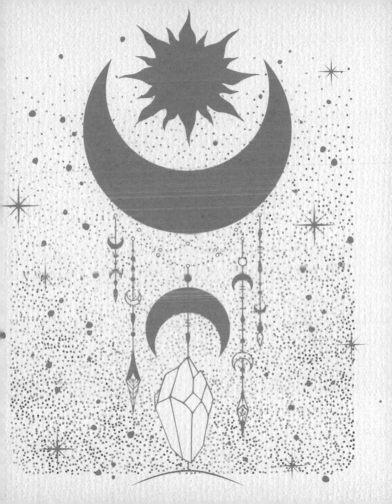

I make the most of the resources I have to help me relax

It's actually a great thing that sleep and sleep quality are now mainstream focuses. There are so many resources available that can help you relax and unwind. One of my favorite resources is music. It's often free, and easily accessible.

Make yourself a relaxation playlist to listen to when you want to unwind. Choose songs that make you feel good and invoke feelings of calm.

Today, I choose to give myself the love, care, and attention I need

Sometimes we look to others to take care of our needs, but it's also important that we don't rely on other people when it's possible for us to meet our needs ourselves.

What needs have you been expecting others to meet when you can meet them yourself?

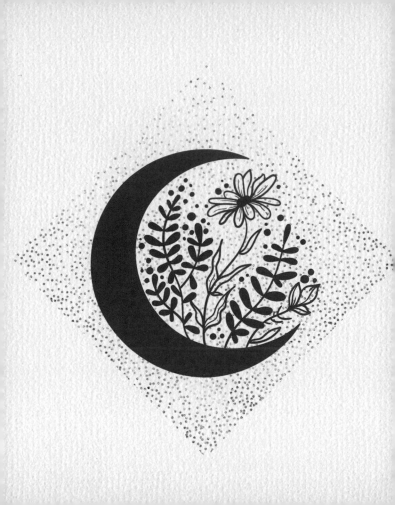

I am enough, exactly as I am in this moment

This is one of my favorite affirmations and probably one of the most powerful of all. There is no truer statement that exists.

Practice saying this affirmation aloud throughout your day and really feel the impact of this statement.

Me time is important to me

We all need alone time, no matter how busy our lives are or how many commitments we have. I used to dread the thought of spending time alone, but now it's something I look forward to. It provides a great opportunity to really get to know yourself.

How does spending time by yourself make you feel?

I listen to the wisdom of my body

There is a lot of wisdom to be found in the constant messages our bodies try to communicate to us. The aches, pains, tightness, or tension might be valuable signs that something needs to change.

What is your body trying to tell you right now about the amount of rest and relaxation it receives?

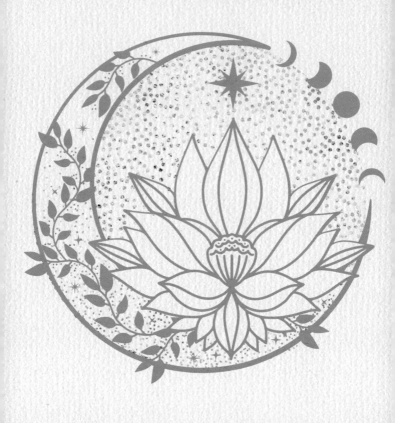

I am a kind, loving, and thoughtful person

Read that again. You don't need me to tell you that you're a good person, but it's nice to be reminded from time to time.

In what ways are you kind, loving, and thoughtful? Journal about a few times you have demonstrated these qualities. If you're struggling with this, ask a trusted loved one about the times you have been there for them.

I tune into my needs on a deeper level than ever before

We might not be aware of our needs until we actually take the time to connect with them. This requires stillness, patience, and a willingness to listen.

Tune into your needs with the following meditation. Get comfortable sitting upright with your spine aligned yet relaxed. Keep your journal close by. Play some soft music if this helps you switch off. Spend a few moments breathing deeply and slowly. When you feel relaxed enough, ask yourself, "What are my needs?" Allow your intuition to answer. You might receive mental pictures, thoughts, or feelings. Spend some time journaling what came up during this meditation.

I move through fear with love, acceptance, and forgiveness

Sometimes fear can be so powerful that it stops you from making any positive changes. Rather than fighting it, see if you can release it with love.

In what ways do you resist or refuse to take care of yourself or look after your needs? Why do you think you do this? Be honest with yourself.

I take care of my needs with gentle and loving energy

You don't need to enforce a strict self-care routine in order to take care of yourself. It is often the smallest changes that have the biggest impact.

How can you be gentler and more loving with yourself on a daily basis?

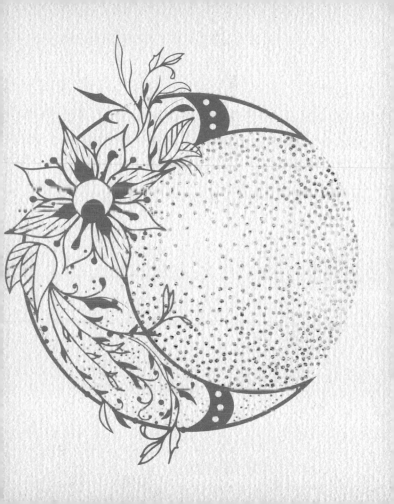

Habit
Changes

Now that we have explored our thoughts and feelings about being worthy of rest, it's time to develop some awareness around our current lifestyle and how we might be able to make small changes that will have a huge impact on our sleep quality.

You begin shaping the quality of your sleep hours before getting into bed. There might be things that you do throughout your day that directly impact the way you will sleep at night. Becoming aware of your current habits and sleep routine is an important part of the journey to cultivating deeper rest and relaxation.

I invite you to be honest with yourself here. In order to make lasting and positive change, we need to be clear on what's currently working and what isn't so effective. This isn't about being critical. Instead, it's about being mindful and taking action to cultivate more effective habits and routines.

Take your time with these affirmations and spend time reflecting on each exercise. If you realize that there are lots of changes you'd like to make, don't panic. Go easy on yourself and start small. As I mentioned earlier, sometimes it's the smallest changes that have the biggest effect. As always, the most important part of the process is being kind to yourself. Enjoy the process and be mindful of how you can cultivate better sleep habits.

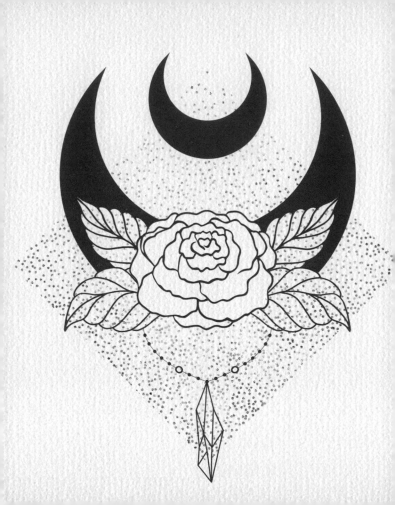

I am willing to make effective changes to my sleep routine

It might seem strange to create a sleep routine, but it's a really effective way of improving your sleep quality. Your sleep routine involves examining what you do one to two hours before you go to bed. Once you have examined your current bedtime routine, you are then in a better place to make healthy changes.

What is your current bedtime routine? How supportive is this to deep and restful sleep?

I am ready to cultivate new habits

Forming a new habit takes time and patience, but the effects can be pretty impressive. Choose one aspect of your bedtime routine to improve for the next thirty days. Make it small and easily achievable.

Keep a habit tracker. Download a habit tracker on your phone or create one in your journal. For every day you complete the task, check off one box. If you're struggling to think of a habit, take inspiration from the following examples: read for twenty minutes in bed before going to sleep, do a ten-minute meditation before sleep, or do stretches and breathing exercises first thing in the morning.

I am excited for all the ways in which I can invite more rest into my life

Making changes can be exciting and enjoyable! If you're feeling overwhelmed at any point, remember that these changes don't have to be drastic. Take it back to the basics and focus on one thing at a time.

What is your favorite healthy way to unwind and relax before you go to bed? Are you currently making enough time for this? If not, is there any way you could make more time for this?

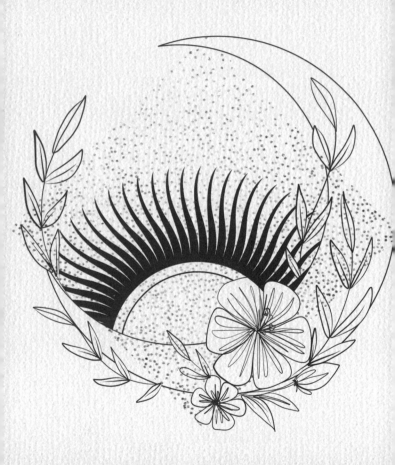

I am honest with myself about what I can change

It takes a level of self-reflection to be honest with yourself about what you are capable of changing. If you're a night owl, then it's best to be realistic about this instead of setting your alarm too early and trying to force yourself to change. Work with your traits, not against them

Complete this sentence: Now that I choose to be honest with myself about what I can change to relax and sleep better, I am going to . . .

I am willing to make positive and lasting changes to my life

In order to make positive and lasting changes to your sleep habits, it's important to know where you're starting from and what already works for you.

Make a list of all the activities, practices, routines, or habits that help you feel calm and peaceful and aid a good night's sleep, then label them in order of most used to least used. Do you have options that you can already draw upon that you haven't made the most out of yet?

I am open to new ways of looking after myself

There may be new practices or techniques out there that could massively benefit your quality of sleep.

What is one wellness or health practice you've always liked the idea of but haven't tried yet? This might include yoga, meditation, massage, or herbal teas. Set yourself a challenge to try this practice and see how it benefits you.

I shape my life in a way that promotes optimum health and happiness

Write down what an average day looks like for you, including as much detail as possible about your routine. Once you have done this, highlight the activities that work well for you. Using another color, highlight the activities that aren't working so well. Rather than feeling overwhelmed if there are several parts of your day that could be improved, choose one aspect and decide to make it your focus.

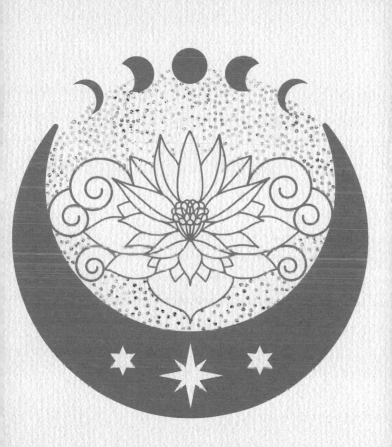

Today I choose to be optimistic about changing my habits

Your initial thoughts and feelings around change might be more negative or pessimistic, and that's okay. Try getting excited about the journey ahead rather than allowing doubt to creep in from day one.

Does making positive change feel possible for you? If the answer is no, why not?

I can do this!

If you struggle with sleep, it might feel like nothing will work and you'll always experience this problem. It can help to think of other areas of life where you've made positive changes.

Make a list of all the ways you have made positive change in the past. How did you feel? What was the trigger for each change?

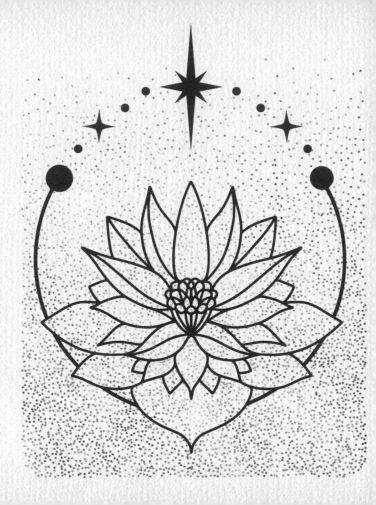

I make changes from a place of self-love

Are you wanting to make changes for yourself, or because you feel like you need to from external sources?

Reflect on why you want to make changes. If you notice your desire to change is not coming from a place of self-love, think about how you can reframe the changes you are making so they are coming from a place of self-love.

I am ready to rest and relax better than I ever have before

You absolutely deserve to experience deep and nourishing sleep, and it is completely possible for you to cultivate more relaxation.

Complete this sentence: Now that I have made the decision to prioritize rest and relaxation, I will . . .

Every tiny change I implement will make a huge difference

Sometimes the small changes to your sleep routine can have a huge impact. Try the following simple change and see how it affects your sleep.

Keep your bedroom a phone-free zone. Charge your phone in another room and use a traditional alarm clock if you need to. This one small change will help you unwind much more easily and will also make your mornings far more peaceful as you wake up without the instant mental stimulation. Or, even better, keep your bedroom an electronics-free zone (remove TVs, iPads, you name it).

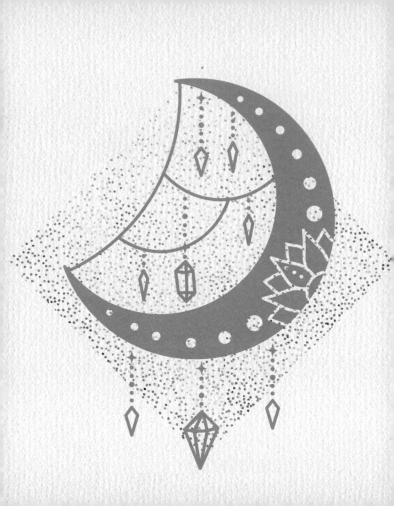

I am always learning and growing

The human experience is one long journey, with each day providing us with a valuable lesson. When we choose to reflect on these lessons with an open mind, change doesn't seem as scary anymore.

Make a list of all the ways you can invite positive change into your life, from small to big changes.

I believe in my ability to make choices supportive of my health and happiness

Deep down, we all want to be healthy and happy. We want to thrive, to feel confident, to show up as our best selves. Self-sabotage comes from a place of fear rather than being what we actually want for ourselves.

Think about your current sleep routine and relaxation practices. In what ways are you self-sabotaging? What is the deeper reason behind why you might do this?

I view my current lifestyle through the lens of loving awareness

This isn't the time to get very critical about yourself and your current lifestyle. Instead, choose to view your current lifestyle from a loving and nonjudgmental frame of mind. Criticizing yourself only keeps you stuck in a negative space.

How much is your current lifestyle prioritizing self-care, relaxation, and deep rest? Why do you think this is?

I am ready to make my well-being a top priority

Hopefully, you are now feeling more comfortable making health a top priority. If you're still feeling some resistance, reflect on where this is coming from and what you can do to shift it.

Make a list of all the ways you would benefit if you decided to make health and well-being a top priority in your life. How would it affect you, your loved ones, and your commitments?

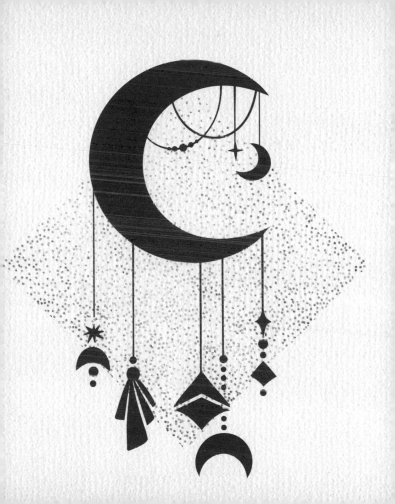

I am more capable than I know

You have faced struggles that you might have thought would break you, but here you still are. You possess a level of resilience that is admirable, and it's time you started giving yourself some credit.

Do you believe it is possible for you to release self-doubt?

I work on myself every day to become a calmer and more relaxed person

If you really want to sleep better and feel peaceful and calm regularly, then it's all about showing up on a daily basis. Working toward something every day shows that you respect yourself and your goals.

If you feel overwhelmed at the idea of working on yourself every single day, don't worry. Create your own definition of what this looks like for you. It might include deleting certain things from your to-do list, or it might include focusing on a general feeling or theme for the day.

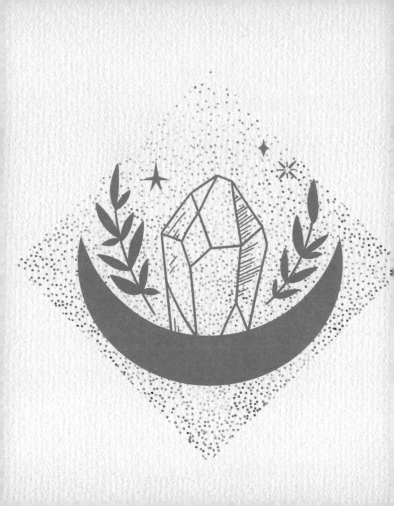

Today I choose
to believe
in myself

Believing in yourself no matter what is a bold move in today's world. We receive so many messages that we aren't enough, so choose to back yourself when others won't. No matter what is going on around you and what other people might say, choose yourself. Do what is best for your well-being, even if it makes others question you. You don't owe anyone an explanation.

Complete this sentence: Choosing to believe in myself for today looks like . . .

I celebrate all my wins, no matter how big or small

Celebrating our achievements shouldn't only be saved for the big things. Get into the habit of acknowledging all of your wins. Even if it's simply making a mental note of something you did well today, it's a good start.

Make a list of all your achievements today, no matter how big or small, that helped you achieve more rest or made you feel proud of yourself.

I am excited to realize my full potential

As you learn more about yourself, implement new sleep habits, and try new tools and techniques, you're proving to yourself that you have so much potential.

Journal about a time in the past—or recently, if you've already begun implementing positive changes—where you connected with your full potential. How did it feel and how did it make you view yourself?

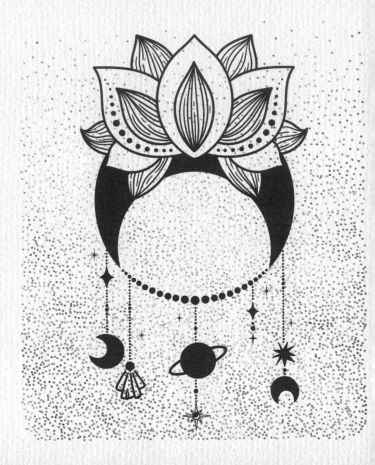

I choose to be kind to myself as I begin to change my habits

Making change can be challenging. There will be days when your new routine or habits fall to the side, and that's okay. It's all about trying again tomorrow and being kind to yourself when things don't go according to plan.

Check in with your current thoughts and feelings. Are you being too critical of yourself? Are you putting too much pressure on yourself? If the answer is yes, consider how you can change your inner dialogue to be more accepting while still maintaining the attitude that change is possible for you.

I am stronger than I realize

Humans have the capacity to endure so much and come out the other side still smiling. We are capable of amazing acts of courage, strength, and bravery.

Try this self-confidence journaling practice. Make a list of all the things you admire, appreciate, or celebrate about yourself. When have you overcome impossible things in the past?

I am motivated, driven, and inspired

Waking up and feeling inspired and motivated is a choice you can decide to make. You are fully capable of choosing this, no matter what you are experiencing.

What is your motivation for making changes to your life for better sleep? What drives you?

As I create new habits, I sleep better than ever

Know that all the habits you're building, the changes you're making, and the limiting beliefs you're challenging will all cumulate in the best sleep you've ever experienced. It might take time to really feel the benefits, but choose to see a good night's sleep as inevitable.

Imagine you've been keeping up with all the positive changes you've been making for at least a few months. What do you imagine you'd feel like? Journal this in as much detail as possible to keep you motivated to make it a reality.

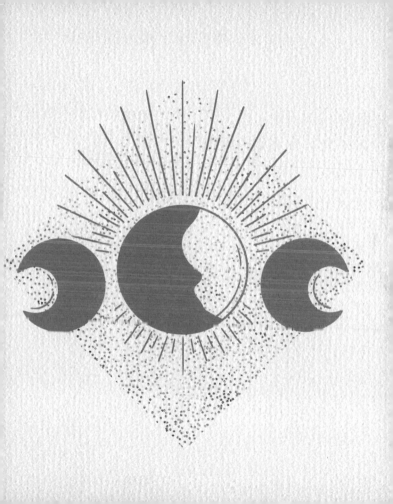

Switch Off
& Relax

A good night's sleep is often directly linked to your ability to switch off and relax. If you find yourself lying in bed thinking about everything from all the tasks you need to get done tomorrow to a strange conversation you had with a friend, it's no secret that you're not going to drift off to sleep anytime soon. Being able to sleep well means you are in a calm and relaxed state, with thoughts no longer going around in circles in your mind.

Switching off is easier said than done, of course, so don't feel frustrated if it takes a while for this to happen, especially if you have a long history with unsettled sleep. Take your time, be patient with yourself, and meet any resistance with compassion and understanding.

The following affirmations and exercises are designed to help you unwind, relax, and switch off from the day. Cultivating calm and inner peace is a great way to fully let go and allow the mind and body to properly rest. You might want to develop a sleep routine that involves keeping this book and your journal next to your bed to use just before you go to sleep or refer to as soon as you wake up in the morning. Allow the calming, peaceful energy of the affirmations to lull you into a deep and restful sleep.

I honor my body's needs and choose to rest more

It takes practice to tune into what your body actually needs, especially when we are so used to living life on autopilot. Your body might have some important messages for you when you take the time to tune in and listen.

Try this body scan meditation before you go to sleep. Get as comfortable as you can lying on your back. Take a few deep, cleansing breaths, exhaling through your mouth to release any tension. Begin to bring your awareness to the top of your head. Allow your awareness to drift through the crown, face, neck, shoulders, arms, hands, chest, abdomen, back, legs, and feet. Direct your awareness to every single part of your body and simply observe any sensations. Don't be surprised if you notice areas of tension you weren't aware of before.

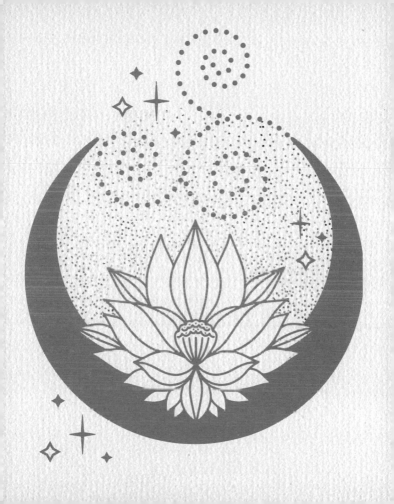

I am ready to let go, rest, and rejuvenate

The simple act of getting your thoughts down on paper will help you begin to switch off before a good night's sleep. It's a good way to get rid of any excess energy that might affect your sleep quality.

Before you get into bed tonight, write down everything that has been playing in your mind. Journal every thought and worry until you feel that you have written them all down. Don't judge it too much or even try to write neatly.

Just for tonight, I let my worries melt away and invite peace into my mind

It can be difficult to give up worries that have become so deeply entrenched. See how the idea of letting your worries go for just one night feels and take it from there.

What does inner peace feel like to you? How does it feel in both your mind and your body?

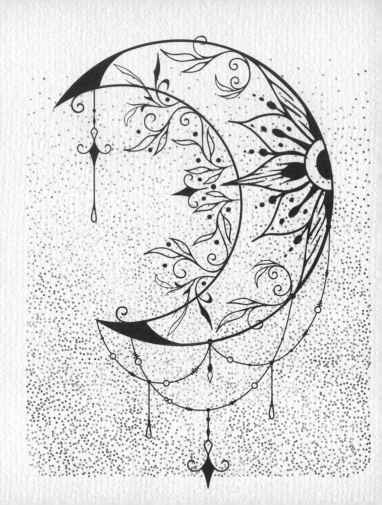

I will create a beautiful and relaxing space to allow myself to rest deeply

Our bedrooms should reflect peace and relaxation. Our environment has a massive impact on our mood, so it's important to create a cozy space that encourages deep rest.

Take some time today to make your bedroom a more peaceful and cozy place. You might consider switching to softer sheets, buying a calming candle, or decluttering your bedside table. Remove anything that doesn't help make the space relaxing. This might include removing electronics as well.

I allow myself to switch off and drift into a deep and relaxing sleep

Sometimes we are unaware of just how much we actually have on our minds. Use this simple exercise to help you mentally prepare for a good night's sleep.

Before you go to bed, visualize the current parts of your life that are taking up lots of energy. It might be a specific person, project, or event. Imagine each item as a light bulb, glowing brightly. Visualize switching off each one before you go to sleep, knowing that you will be even more refreshed in the morning to begin working on them again.

I am ready to refresh, repair, and restore my body and mind

The less stimulation we have in the hours before sleep, the better. Stimulating activities include watching intense films or TV shows, checking social media, or anything else that involves using technology that energizes the mind rather than relaxing it.

Try a technology-free hour before bedtime. Switch off the TV, place your phone on silent, and spend the time winding down. You might wish to have a long and relaxing shower, read a book, or make a cup of caffeine-free tea.

I welcome a good night's sleep with gratitude and appreciation

You might be in the habit of thinking about your current stresses and worries before you go to sleep, but how about challenging this and forming a new habit of practicing gratitude instead?

Practice bedtime gratitude. Journal, speak aloud, or think of a few things that you're grateful for. Focus on the good things that happened in your day. If you share your bed, consider doing this practice with your partner.

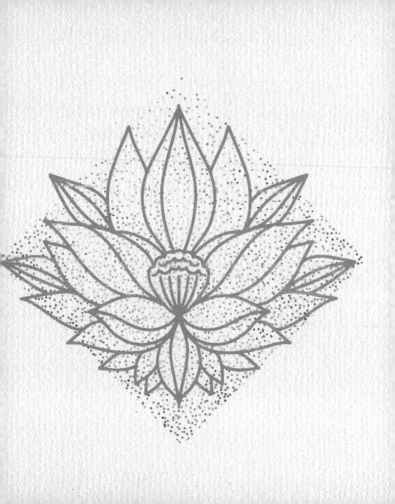

All is well and I am completely supported

A big part of not being able to switch off and sleep well is caused by the attitude that we must be "on" 24/7, and that rest will actually hinder us in some way. Here's a revolutionary idea: the world will not fall to pieces if you take your foot off the pedal for the night. Support is available to you.

Who or what helps you feel safe and supported? How can they help you achieve more rest?

I embrace the stillness

When we have long or intense conversations before sleep, it increases mental activity, which makes it difficult to switch off. This includes any phone calls or text conversations. Focus on making your evening as relaxing as possible.

To help you switch off, try spending some time before you go to bed free of any conversations. If you live with loved ones, try making an agreement to have some quiet time before bed. Even if it's only five minutes, it will help you relax.

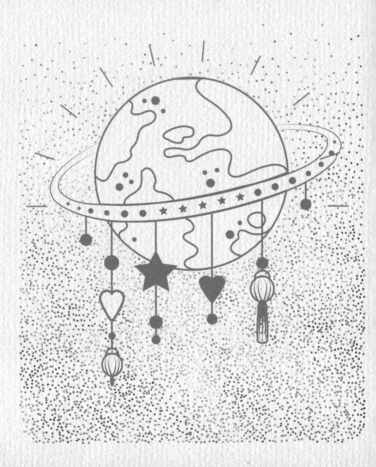

I give myself permission to receive deep rest

Mentally giving ourselves permission for deep rest helps communicate to the body that changes are going to take place. We are what we repeatedly tell ourselves, so see what happens when you grant yourself that permission.

Complete this sentence: Now that I have given myself permission to let go and fully rest, I feel . . .

I invite peaceful and relaxing energy into every single cell of my body

You can make the decision to invite more peace into your body. It is completely within your power to call this energy into every single part of you.

Practice this peaceful color meditation to help invite more calming energy into your nightly routine. As you drift off to sleep, visualize scanning your body with a beautiful healing light of your color choice. Allow this light to cover every inch of your body, infusing you with a nourishing and restorative energy. Direct this light longer on areas that need it most.

I inhale calmness and exhale pressure

The breath is a powerful tool that is always available to us. Use this nervous system-regulation breathing technique to release any pressure in your body before bed and induce a calm feeling. Breathe in, then out, keeping your exhales longer than your inhales. Making your exhales longer than your inhales can positively affect the vagus nerve, which is associated with encouraging rest and relaxation. Allow your body to guide you as you breathe. Only do what feels comfortable and do not try to force the breath.

As I quiet my mind, I allow my body to naturally balance and release tension

Your body is an amazing creation. There are trillions of cells working tirelessly to keep you alive and healthy right now in this moment.

Write down five things you are grateful for about your body.

With every breath, I become more and more relaxed

This affirmation can have a hypnotic effect when practiced alongside mindful breathing exercises. Allow this affirmation to lull you into a state of pure relaxation.

Repeat this affirmation to yourself with every intentional breath. Close your eyes and allow your breath to guide you as you relax more and more.

I am calm,
I am balanced,
I am at peace

Taking time to balance and calm your body naturally balances and calms your mind. Slow and gentle movements have the capacity to relax you without having to think too much.

Before you go to bed, do some stretches to help you calm your body. Take a few gentle stretches either next to or on your bed. You can stretch in any way that feels good or find an online video to follow for guidance. Focus on slow, relaxing, gentle postures. Make sure you don't get your heart rate up and the postures help you unwind.

I receive guidance and wisdom through my dreams

Often our subconscious is trying to communicate to us through the medium of dreams, if only we are willing to listen. Our dreams can provide us with many messages and clues.

Keep a dream journal next to your bed and write down your dreams as soon as you wake up. Do you notice any messages or clues? What might your subconscious be trying to tell you?

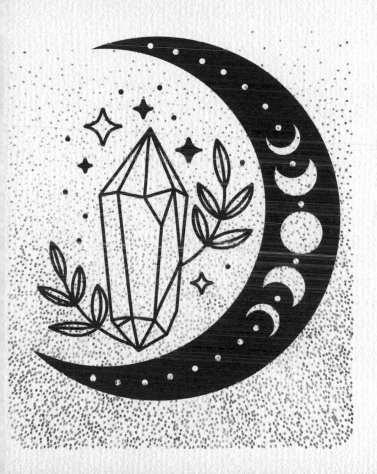

I did my best today, and now I am ready to recharge

Doing your best is much better than doing something perfectly. It's okay if something didn't work out as you had hoped; if you tried your best, then that's all that really matters.

How did you try your best today? Why should you be proud of yourself for this?

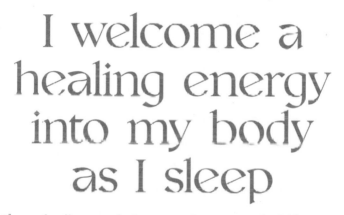

I welcome a healing energy into my body as I sleep

Place a healing or calming quotation on your bedside table or somewhere you can see it near your bed so you are reminded of it every time you get into bed. You might wish to write your favorite affirmations instead and place them where you can see them. Read them every time you go to sleep.

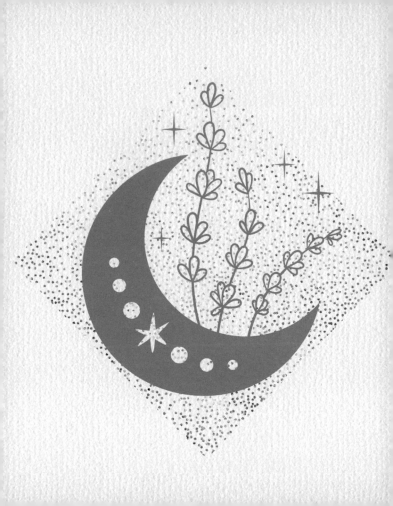

I let go of
the day

The following closing tabs visualization technique might
seem a little strange, but I promise you it's very effective.
I have practiced this for years and it never fails to make
me feel calmer!

As you get into bed and feel yourself begin to relax,
picture an internet browser screen with lots of tabs
open. Imagine each tab is an aspect of your life. Visualize
yourself clicking off each tab, closing down any remaining
thoughts or worries you might have. Keep closing them
down until none remain.

It is natural and easy for me to sleep well

The human body is designed to thrive. It knows exactly what to do to regenerate and repair. You don't have to tell your liver to detoxify; it simply does it.

What negative beliefs do you still hold around your capacity to switch off and rest well? Spend some time journaling any resistance or limiting thoughts you might have around this.

I wake up feeling deeply rested and ready for a fulfilling new day

How we spend the morning has a big impact on the quality of the day, and even that night's sleep. Even a simple five-minute morning routine will make a difference.

How do you currently spend the first half hour to an hour of your day? Journal your current habits and routines. Once you have done this, be honest with yourself and see whether there is anything you could change to make this time more beneficial to your health and well-being.

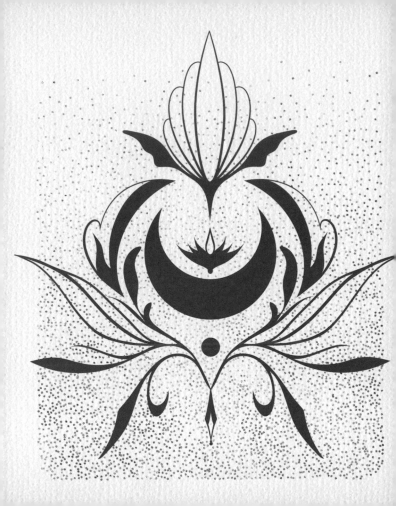

I am safe and settled

We often take our physical surroundings for granted. If you woke up this morning in a safe space, including a comfy bed, with a roof over your head, you are more fortunate than a good proportion of the world.

What do you like the most about your physical surroundings? What items help you feel comfy, relaxed, and peaceful?

For tonight, I let go of my troubles and sleep peacefully

Your worries do not require you to think about them all the time. Even if you have a complex problem that needs solving, you can't spend all your time thinking about it. Sleeping is actually a really good way to help solve your problems, because you will wake up with a fresh mind and more energy in the morning.

Choose two or three issues that have been playing on your mind recently and write them down in your journal. Once you have done this, answer the following questions: I am grateful for this experience because . . . The biggest lesson I am learning from this experience is . . . I can choose to see this situation differently by . . .

I invite all aspects of myself to return to a state of balance

We spend our days in so many different locations, speaking to many different people and viewing so much content on our devices. This can leave our energy feeling scattered.

Practice this bedtime visualization to calm your energy. Before you go to sleep, visualize where you have been throughout the day, the people you have spoken to, and the things that have taken your attention. Imagine yourself calling back your energy from these situations, so it returns to you. I visualize this as a golden energy rushing back into my body. It helps me sleep better knowing that all of my energy has now returned to me.

I give thanks for the gift of a new day

Waking up in the morning is the most beautiful gift of all. You have the opportunity to experience life and all of its lessons, to love your family and friends, to make a real difference on this planet.

As soon as you wake up in the morning, before you open your eyes, repeat this affirmation, either aloud or in your mind. Starting your day with gratitude is a great way to increase feelings of appreciation.

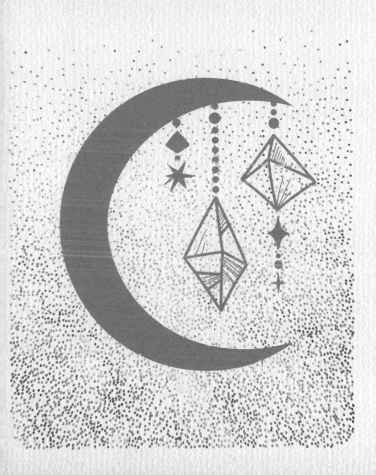

Release
Pressure &
Expectations

So far, we have worked to increase worthiness around rest and relaxation, mindfully examined our current sleep habits and routines, and empowered ourselves with the ability to switch off and relax. The final step in getting a good night's sleep involves releasing any pressure and expectations you place on yourself around being able to sleep well.

We've all been there—lying in bed, watching the clock tick away, or staring into the darkness, feeling so unsettled, and noticing frustration and tension beginning to rise. It's not a nice feeling, and the more frustrated you feel, the further away sleep seems. The following affirmations and exercises are designed to help you release any tension or pressure that builds up around not being able to sleep well.

Sleep isn't something that we check off our to-do lists or receive a grade for. Life is unpredictable and messy at the best of times. There will be some nights when, for whatever reason, you won't get as much sleep as you'd like, and that is perfectly okay. The sun will still rise in the morning, and you will get the opportunity to sleep better tomorrow. The goal of this chapter is to help ease some of the tension during these nights when it might be hard to get to sleep. Allow these affirmations and exercises to help you get some rest.

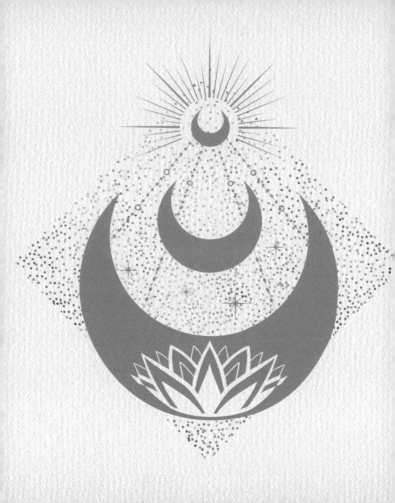

I release what I cannot control and trust that all is well

There are so many factors in life that are beyond our control. The sooner we accept this, the sooner we can make peace with the unpredictable nature of life.

What circumstances are you holding on to that are truly out of your control and cannot be influenced by you? Journal all the ways in which you have been holding on to these things.

There is nothing for me to do apart from rest and relax

Sometimes when we get into bed and our mind settles, we are reminded of the many tasks we need to complete or things we need to work on.

Instead of spending the night thinking about these things, grab your journal and make a list of everything that is on your mind. Once you have done this, cross out each one and write next to it, "This is not my job for tonight. I choose to let it go."

I aim for contentment rather than certainty

When you get into bed each night, you can't be certain that you'll sleep perfectly. In fact, you can't be certain about most things, but you can definitely choose to be content with whatever does or doesn't happen.

What does contentment feel like for you? Write down your own definition in your journal and make a list of all the things that help strengthen this feeling.

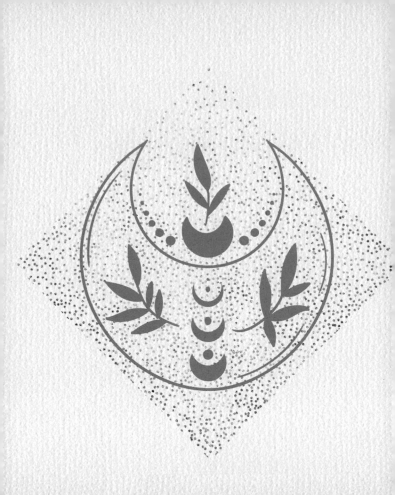

I accept both good and bad nights and go with the flow

Nature is always flowing and moving without effort or thought. If we allow ourselves to, we can also experience this flow, without getting caught up in the things that damage our peace.

Try this exercise to help you allow more flow into your life. If you live near a river or body of water, try spending some time today observing how the water flows without effort. If you don't live near water, watch some online videos of waterfalls, rivers, the sea, or anything else that feels right. Let the peaceful waves wash over you, knowing that nature is flowing all around you without any control or effort.

I am peaceful, knowing that the sun will rise again tomorrow

Know that as the sun rises every morning, you will also continue to rise, even when things seem dark or uncertain.

Practice this rising sun visualization for a few minutes before bed. Relax your body, either sitting upright or lying down, and turn your attention inward. Slow and deepen your breath and let yourself arrive in the moment. Imagine a dark sky somewhere in nature. See the sky gradually changing color from black to hints of orange, red, and yellow. Visualize the sun rising on the horizon, illuminating the sky with golden light. Breathe in this beautiful awakening energy, focusing on feelings of renewal and hope.

I quiet the part of myself that worries at bedtime

If you struggle with sleep, it's easy to jump to the conclusion that every single night is the same for you, and it can be very hard to stop worrying. However, if you think long enough, you might be able to recall times when you did sleep well. Remind yourself of these experiences rather than letting worry take over.

Think about the last time you slept really well. Where were you? How did you feel in the morning? How did it impact your day? Focusing on this memory will help you remember just how important a good night's sleep is and that it is absolutely possible to replicate because you've already done it.

I stop putting so much pressure on myself and accept myself exactly as I am

You already face enough pressure from family, friends, colleagues, and society without putting even more pressure on yourself. Give yourself a break. You deserve it.

What is the biggest pressure you put on yourself and where did you learn to do this?

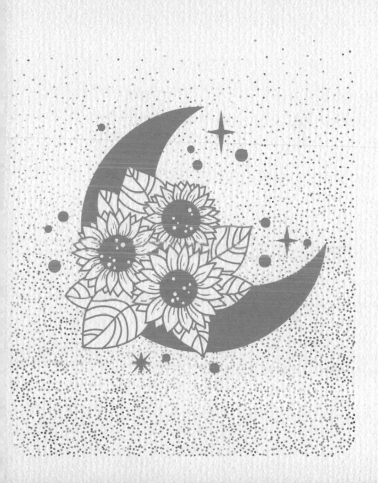

I let go of the expectations others place on me

We all place expectations on others, whether we are aware of it or not. This can amount to a lot of pressure to carry and can impact the way we see ourselves.

Who are you currently feeling pressure from? What expectations do you feel they are trying to make you meet? How does this make you feel? What is the healthiest way to release these expectations?

I meet frustration with kindness and understanding

It's okay to feel annoyance and frustration toward ourselves. The key is not letting these feelings develop into criticism, which we then internalize. You get to decide how to process these thoughts and feelings. Rather than believing them to be true, is it possible to question them and choose more helpful thoughts or feelings?

Complete this sentence: Instead of getting frustrated with myself, I choose to . . .

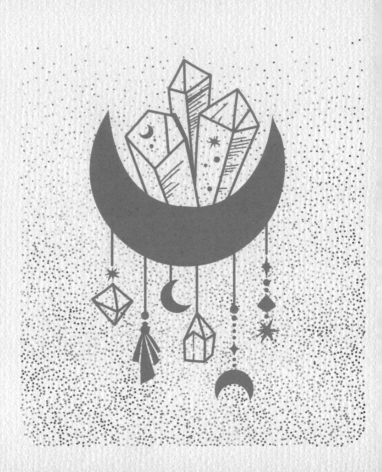

As I climb into bed tonight, I leave the past behind me

Shining a light on our past experiences means we can begin to process them so they no longer have an effect on us in the present day. We can't change the past, but we can change how we view our past experiences.

What past experiences do you carry around that still affect you to this day? Write them down and explore how they still make you feel. Meet any feelings with loving kindness. You aren't trying to change what happened; you are simply bringing awareness to how you still carry the experience with you. Don't put pressure on yourself for the feelings to disappear after one journaling session. You might wish to work through any difficult memories or feelings with a health care professional.

I shake away any excess energy from the day

Sometimes all that's needed is a big release of stored-up energy. Our bodies can store years of tension without us even realizing it.

Add this exercise to your nighttime routine. Take a few minutes to shake your body in any way that feels good. Shake your legs, arms, head, hands, and anything else that feels tense. Inhale deeply, then exhale loudly as you do this and feel any tension or unprocessed emotions begin to dissolve. Shaking your body also helps burn off excess adrenaline, which will help you relax before bedtime.

I replace worry with inner peace

Explore your options before you respond to worry. There might be lots of different actions you can take. Pausing before you act can help you arrive at the right decision.

Write down the most prominent worries you are currently thinking about. For each one, write down something you could think, do, or say that would help you feel more inner peace about the situation.

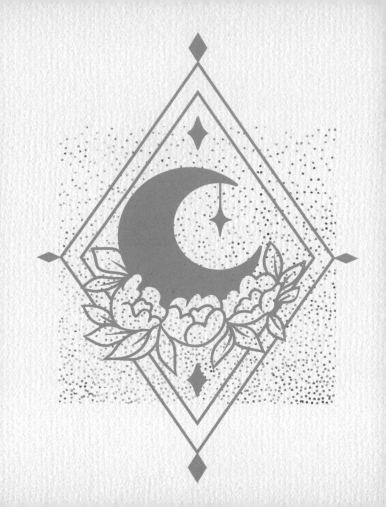

I invite my intuition to communicate with me through my dreams

Allow your intuition to communicate to you in ways you might have not considered before.

Take a piece of paper and write down something you would like to receive clarification or answers about. Make a mental note to receive answers through your dreams. Place this piece of paper under your pillow as you sleep. When you wake up, take this piece of paper and begin writing down any dreams you had during the night. See whether you can make any connections to your question. Remember, dreams are often symbolic, so the meaning may not be so literal.

As I sleep, I invite my mind to shed any limiting beliefs or patterns

Our subconscious mind governs most of our brain activity, and yet we aren't even aware of this. You can, however, give your subconscious mind instructions that can benefit you.

Practice this "walking down the stairs" visualization. As you get comfortable in bed and close your eyes, feel your whole body relax and let go. While you slow your breathing and feel even more peaceful, visualize a staircase before you. Take a deep breath and take the first step down. Continue to do this, counting down from ten as you take another step, dropping deeper and deeper into relaxation. Once you reach one, ask yourself, "What does my subconscious need to show me?"

I welcome the possibility of making peace with exactly where I am

We are often so quick to race ahead to our goals that the present moment slips right past us. There could be some valuable lessons to experience exactly where you are, if only you stopped to look.

Take a few minutes to write your answers to the following questions in your journal or a separate piece of paper. What if where you are right now in life is exactly where you need to be? What if all the obstacles or issues you're facing are exactly what you need for optimal growth?

No matter what I experience, I can and will get through it

Even if you experience the worst insomnia, restlessness, or stress, know that eventually it will pass. You can't predict how or when, but try to take comfort in the fact that it will.

Think about a time when you experienced something you thought you'd never recover from but did. How did you manage to get through it? What lessons did you learn about yourself?

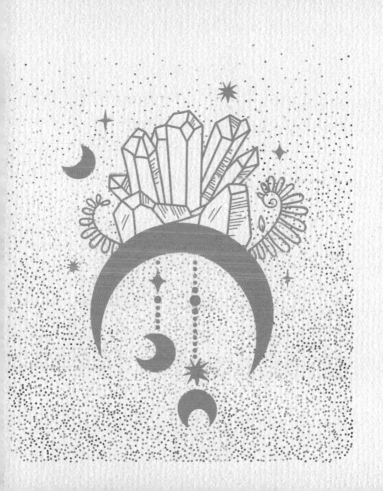

I live in harmony with my mind, my body, my loved ones, and my surroundings

To live in harmony means to go with the flow of life, even when things happen out of the blue. Rather than resisting unexpected changes (which leads to more stress and tension), try moving toward peace instead, trusting that you're strong enough to endure any direction your life moves in.

In what ways are you out of harmony with your mind, body, loved ones, and surroundings? What actions can you take to invite more harmony into your life?

I choose to experience sleep rather than try to accomplish it

Good sleep is so much more than a goal or an activity you can improve. You can, of course, work to establish new habits and routines around sleep, but at the end of the day, sleep is there to be experienced.

In what ways have you been viewing sleep as something you need to do or accomplish rather than experience?

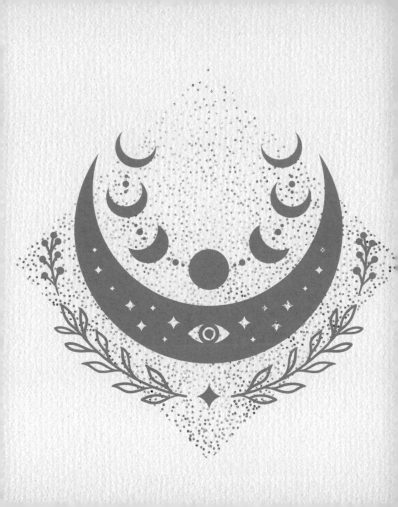

There is nothing for me to do apart from inviting feelings of rest into my mind and body

Bedtime is not the time to worry and fret. It is literally time to be in your bed. There is no other purpose to this moment apart from resting and relaxing.

Write your answers to the following question in your journal or on a separate piece of paper. What would you really achieve by worrying about all the things you have to do tomorrow as you try to sleep?

I let my anxiety melt away with ease

Anxiety is not something that easily goes away. Often, the best we can do is give our anxiety some acknowledgment and love, then spend time trying to release those anxious feelings. Don't be scared of your anxiety. It's here to teach you something, not to punish you.

Try this visualization exercise a few minutes before bed to help you release your anxiety and get your body ready for rest. Get comfortable on your bed, supporting your head and placing a pillow under your knees if this feels good for you. Check in with your body. Where do you notice any feelings of anxiety, tension, or nervousness? Locate the places within your body. Visualize the energy from these places begin to melt and dissipate into the surface beneath you. You might want to visualize this energy as heavy and sticky, slowly melting and leaving your body with every breath.

No matter what I think or feel, I always choose to forgive myself

Forgiveness is one of the biggest keys to a peaceful life. Forgive others, but most importantly, forgive yourself. What do you need to forgive yourself for?

Every night is an opportunity for me to move in a better direction

You are doing so well, and you should feel so proud of yourself for how far you've come. Don't give up now!

What positive changes have you made recently that are helping you move in the right direction?

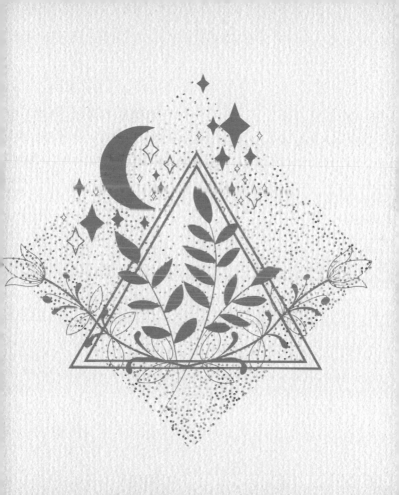

I settle into a silent and supportive sleep

Amazing insight can be found in silence, yet we rarely experience it in today's busy world. When was the last time you experienced silence?

Take some time today or this evening to be silent. Turn off all electrical devices, stop all music from playing, and simply be present in the stillness.

I respect my body's signals for more rest and relaxation

Your body really does know best. Do you feel like sleeping in a little longer and have the option to do so? Listen to those signals and let yourself rest. Respect the wisdom of your body.

Try sleeping without an alarm on the days you're able to. Let yourself wake up naturally at whatever time feels right. If you lead a busy life and this isn't possible, try finding ten or fifteen minutes during the day when you can sit or lie down, rest, or even nap.

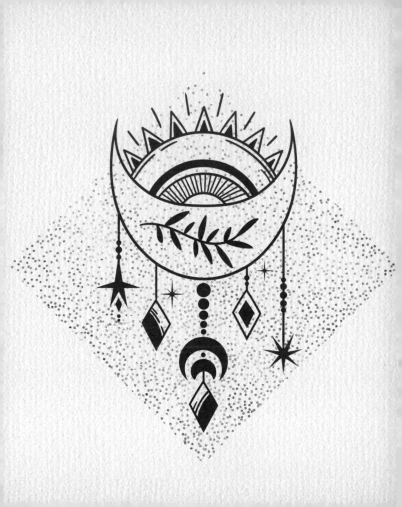

I drift off into a peaceful sleep with a settled mind and a grateful heart

Whether you've just begun your journey to better sleep or you've been on this path for quite some time, congratulate yourself. You have chosen to make big and small changes, which all require a lot of courage. Be proud of yourself!

Make a list of all your achievements and breakthroughs, no matter how big or small, and place it somewhere you will see it. Whenever you next feel doubtful or unsettled, refer back to this list.

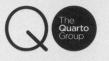

Q The Quarto Group

Inspiring | Educating | Creating | Entertaining

Brimming with creative inspiration, how-to projects, and useful information to enrich your everyday life, quarto.com is a favorite destination for those pursuing their interests and passions.

First published in 2023 by Rock Point, an imprint of The Quarto Group, 142 West 36th Street, 4th Floor, New York, NY 10018, USA
T (212) 779-4972 F (212) 779-6058 www.Quarto.com

Rock Point titles are also available at discount for retail, wholesale, promotional, and bulk purchase. For details, contact the Special Sales Manager by email at specialsales@quarto.com or by mail at The Quarto Group, Attn: Special Sales Manager, 100 Cummings Center Suite 265D, Beverly, MA 01915 USA.

10 9 8 7 6 5 4 3 2 1

ISBN: 978-1-63106-867-6

Printed in China

Library of Congress Cataloging-in-Publication Data

Names: Trewick, Elicia Rose, author.
Title: Dreams: 100 affirmations for a good night's sleep / Elicia Rose Trewick.
Other titles: Dreams: one hundred affirmations for a good night's sleep
Description: New York, NY : Rock Point, 2022. | Series: Inspiring guides |
  Summary: "Getting enough rest at night is made easy and simple with
  Dreams: 100 Affirmations for a Good Night's Sleep, your bedtime ritual
  filled with affirmations and guided prompts to help you achieve personal
  growth"—Provided by publisher.
Identifiers: LCCN 2021061824 (print) | LCCN 2021061825 (ebook) | ISBN
  9781631068676 (hardcover) | ISBN 9780760376393 (ebook)
Subjects: LCSH: Sleep. | Dreams. | Affirmations.
Classification: LCC RA786 .T74 2022 (print) | LCC RA786 (ebook) | DDC
  612.8/21--dc23/eng/20220211
LC record available at https://lccn.loc.gov/2021061824
LC ebook record available at https://lccn.loc.gov/2021061825

Publisher: Rage Kindelsperger   Editor: Keyla Pizarro-Hernández
Creative Director: Laura Drew   Cover and Interior Design: Amy Sly
Managing Editor: Cara Donaldson

About the Author

Elicia Rose is a writer and illustrator based in Sheffield, England. She is the creator of Bloom Affirmations. What originally began as an Instagram page trying to make social media a kinder place to be has bloomed into an array of work, all focused on helping people feel better about themselves through the power of positive affirmations. Find out more at bloomaffirmations.com